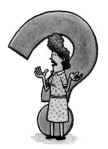

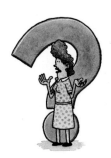

# WHAT'S *stopped*^

## by Dale Burg

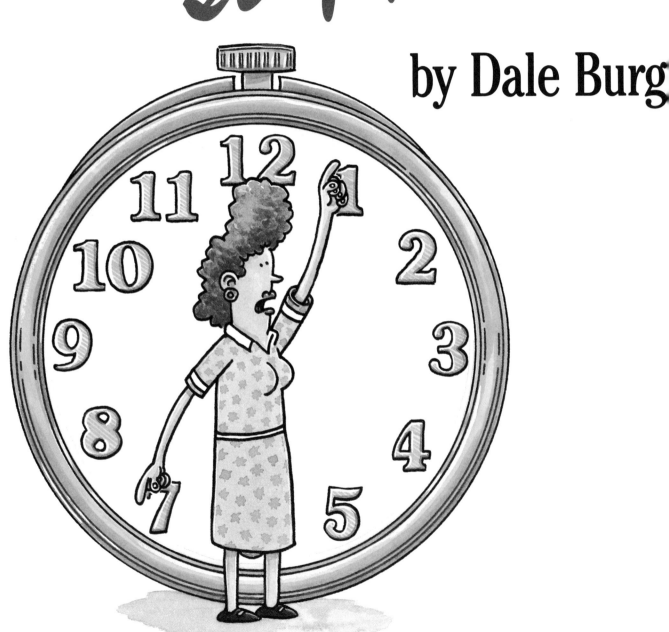

# HAPPENING TO ME?

with Mary Jane Minkin, M.D.

Illustrated by John Kerschbaum

A Citadel Press Book
Published by Carol Publishing Group

Carol Publishing Group Edition - 1993

A Citadel Press Book
Published by Carol Publishing Group
Citadel Press  is a registered trademark of Carol Publishing Group

Editorial Offices:  600 Madison Avenue, New York, NY 10022
Sales & Distribution Offices:  120 Enterprise Avenue, Secaucus, NJ  07094
In Canada: Canadian Manda Group, P.O. Box 920, Station U, Toronto,
Ontario, M8Z 5P9, Canada

Queries regarding rights and permissions should be addressed to:
Carol Publishing Group, 600 Madison Avenue, New York, NY 10022

Manufactured in the United States of America
ISBN 0-8065-1417-5

Carol Publishing Group books are available at special discounts
for bulk purchases, for sales promotions, fund raising, or
educational purposes.  Special editions can also be created to
specifications.  For details contact: Special Sales Department,
Carol Publishing Group, 120 Enterprise Ave., Secaucus,  NJ  07094

Library of Congress Cataloging-in-Publication Data

Burg, Dale.
      "What's stopped happening to me?" / by Dale Burg  and Mary Jane
   Minkin ; illustrated by John Kerschbaum.
        p.  cm.
      "A Citadel Press Book"
      1. Menopause.  I. Minkin, Mary Jane.  II. Title.
   RG186.B83   1990                        90-41896
      612.6'65—dc20                         CIP

For every woman
who read
**WHAT'S HAPPENING
TO ME?**
to find out about
puberty.
And for every woman
who didn't.

*If you're* **40** *this one's*
*over* *for you*

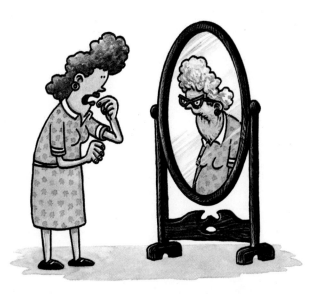

## The Acknowledgments
## From Mary Jane

Bonnie, Dawn, Debbie,
..............
Edwina, Isabel, Jill,
..............
Joyce, Julie, Kathy,
..............
Kris, Mary Lake,
..............
Randy, Rhea,
..............
Roberta, Rose, Shirley,
..............
Stephanie, Vivian,
..............
Mother

..............................................

# The Acknowledgments
## From Dale

Abby, Alice, Ann,

Bambe, Barbara, Bonnie,

Carol, Connie, Cynthia,

Darlene, Dorothy,

Elaine, Faye, Gail, Gay,

Harriet, Hattie, Helen, Helene,

Jane Elise, Jill, Joyce,

Karen, Katie, Linda,

Margot, Marilyn, Mary, Mary Ellen,

Meredith, Mother, Myrna, Myra,

Laurette, Nancy, Pam, Patty, Paula,

Rita, Sandy, Seena, Susan, Sue, Suzy, Sybil,

Tanya, Teddi, Trish, Vicki

......and all others

# CONT

# E N T S

# They try to tell you that hitting forty is no big deal.

*T*hat's true. Compared to, say, finding out that your husband is being transferred to Bangladesh; that your son, the college student, wants to become a mime; or that your mother is divorcing your father to run off with her dance instructor, it's nothing.

There are some things you *can* do about getting older. Aerobics. Sunscreens. Control-top stockings. But you know, and we know, that even if they're still asking for your ID in bars, it's coming.

Menopause. The Big M.

It is possible that one of your friends has personal knowledge of what it's like. Don't count on her to share it. This is one of the few areas in which everyone is competing to be last.

Women who will confide all the details of their collagen injections and tell you exactly where they get their designer clothes at discount keep their lips buttoned when it comes to menopause. It's the only detail that the "tell-all" books never tell.

So where do you get your information? If you want to read a book about menstruation, you can find a lot of books that treat it like one of the diseases of old age. (As if you didn't have enough problems just adjusting to your new bifocals.)

We figured you're like us. You wanted to know what's going on in your body. Not enough to depress you, but enough to give you the general idea. That's why we wrote this book.

It may not answer all your questions or solve all your problems. But when you're through reading it, you should know a lot more about what will happen — or will stop happening — to you.

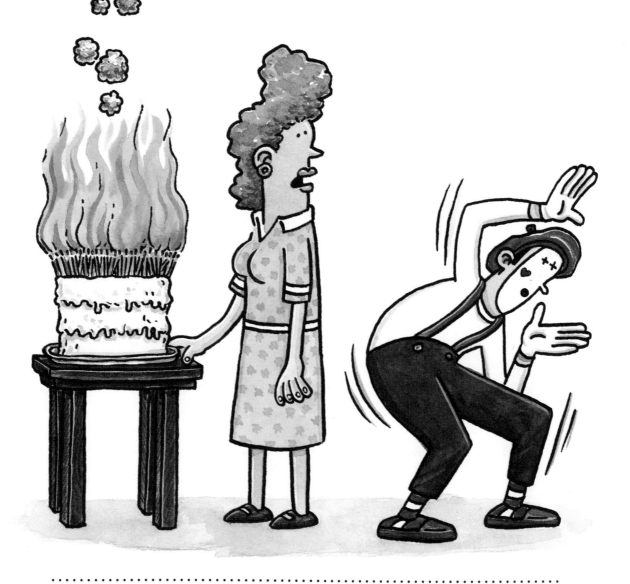

# "Does this happen
...................................
# to everyone?"

*N*o. It does not happen to men. It does, however, happen to all women.

And, it's a safe assumption that it has already happened to Ursula Andress, all the Gabors and Jackie O. Not to mention Margaret Thatcher. They all seem to be doing well and looking good. No reason you can't either.

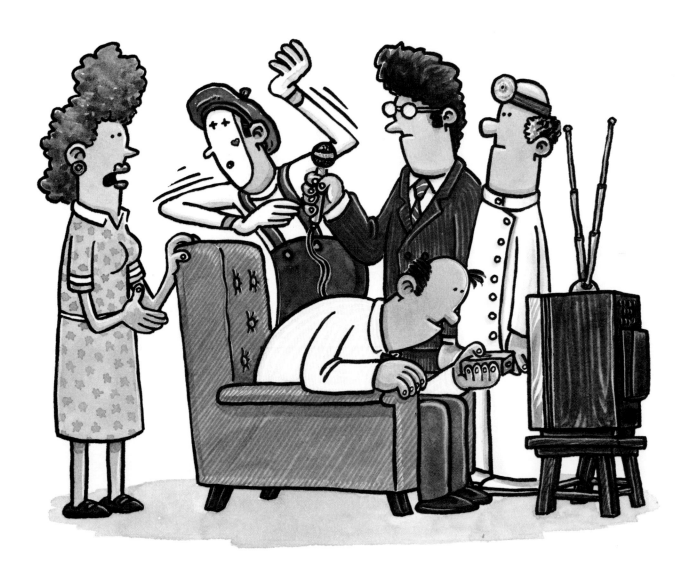

# When it happens.

*I*t can happen as early as 35 and even later than 58. One out of ten women starts by age 40. Most women reach menopause by age 50 or 51.

At the turn of the century, women didn't have to worry about things like pension plans, empty nesting and menopause. They didn't live long enough. The average life expectancy was only 48.

There seems to be no correlation between whether you were "late" or "early" in beginning to menstruate, whether or not you took birth control pills, or whether or not you were an early reader.

The only thing that does seem to matter is when your mother and/or other female relatives reached menopause. Chances are, if they were early, you will be too.

Although you may have said to yourself many times that you would NEVER do what your mother did, this is yet another case in which you probably will.

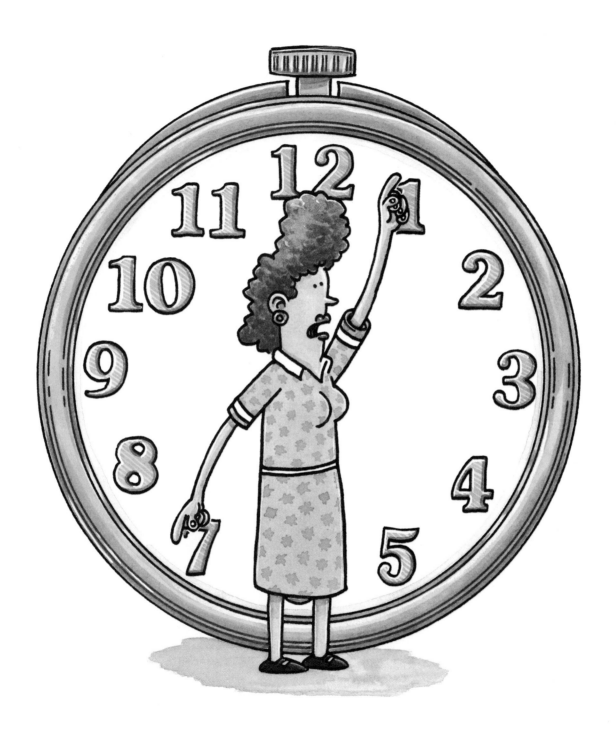

# Why it happens.

........................

*M*enopause is ovary burnout. The ovaries, which store egg cells, also manufacture the hormone estrogen. Estrogen is responsible for the major female characteristics: high voice, breast development, and (some say) an interest in flea marketing. It also helps develop and maintain many body tissues, particularly those of the breasts, bones, skin, bladder and vagina.

You are born with a lifetime supply of egg cells, but by the time you reach puberty, you've already lost half of them. (This is true even if you're one of those organization freaks who never loses anything.)

During each cycle, 20 to 1,000 eggs mature (though only one is generally released into the fallopian tubes each month). Eventually, when there are no eggs left, you no longer menstruate.

**Though men don't get around to producing sperm until they reach puberty, a girl is born with about 700,000 eggs. (Women's bodies plan ahead. Men's don't. Isn't that typical?)**

●

........................

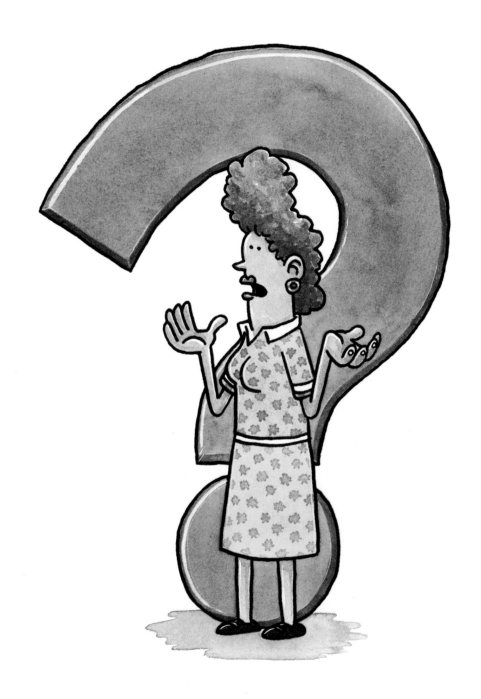

# "How will I know when menopause has started?"

*H*ere are some milestones that might indicate it's coming:

Your gynecologist/lawyer/accountant (pick one or all) is now younger than you are.

You go to the movies and find yourself attracted to the male lead with gray temples instead of the young one.

You notice that these days, when you're lying on your side, your stomach is lying on its stomach.

Medically, however, none of these count.

According to a doctor, the only reliable indicator that you're what is officially called "perimenopausal" is that your cycles have become irregular and your bleeding is heavier.

The cycles are irregular because some months you won't ovulate. Your periods may be as close together as 14 days or as far apart as 56. (Late periods at this age may cause a certain amount of confusion. You may not be sure whether to start buying smaller boxes of tampons or a pregnancy testing kit.)

There is more bleeding because your progesterone levels, like your estrogen levels, are going down. (There are blood tests to check hormone levels but they are not very reliable. The levels change almost as often as your husband switches TV channels.)

Spotting may be a sign of menopause but also may indicate other problems. See your doctor. But clots (which are no cause for concern) are common. (Wouldn't you rather have a D flawless diamond, which is rare?)

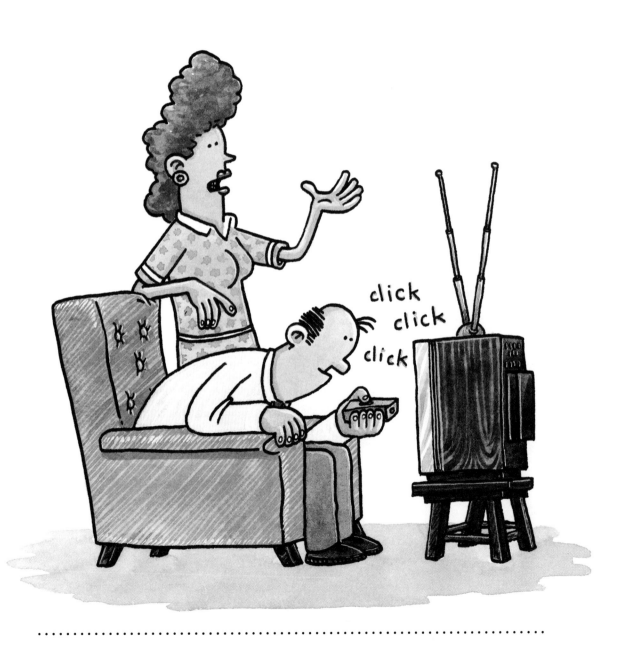

# "When does it end?"

*T*he only way to know it's over is when you have gone a year without your period. That's when you throw away the overnight pads and the super tampons. Not until then can you throw away the contraceptives as well. (Ignore this rule only if you like surprises that can be diapered.)

Imagine what you will be able to do with all that extra room in your nighttable.

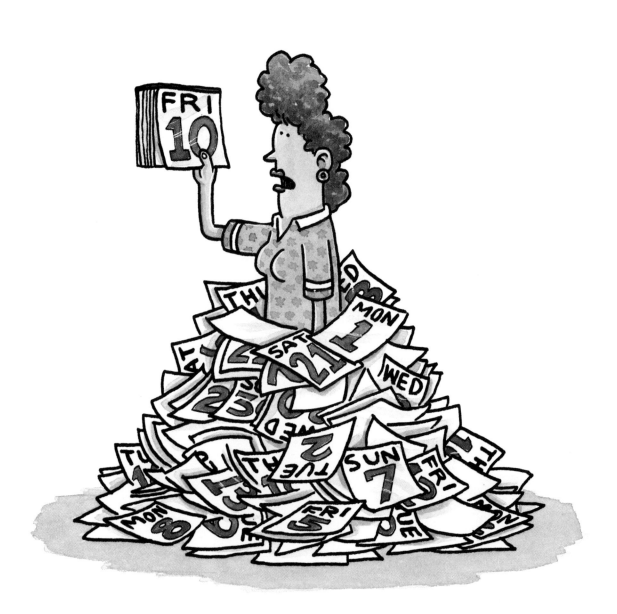

# "Will I get
# fat/old/depressed
# immediately?"

*T*hough your periods have become irregular, that does not mean that one morning you will wake up and see an overweight, unhappy hag looking back from your bathroom mirror (unless, of course, you saw her in the mirror the night before).

Good news: Gaining weight is not a symptom of menopause.

Bad news: Gaining weight is a symptom of aging. Your basal metabolism goes down. Unfortunately, left to its own devices your appetite will completely ignore this development.

As for the other symptoms, they occur gradually. Many women are hardly troubled by them. Some skip them completely: they're menstruating regularly and then — all of a sudden — it's gone. (You will recognize this pattern from many past dating experiences.)

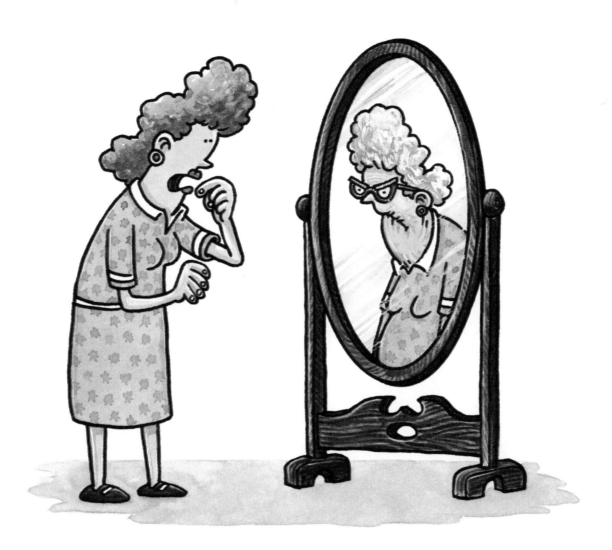

# "Will I act weird?"

*T*his is like asking, "Will I be able to play the piano after the operation?" Could you play it before?

You may, in fact, act a little strange. Your estrogen level is going down, and estrogen helps increase the blood flow to the brain. No one knows for sure if that affects your memory. Middle-aged men, who've never had estrogen, become forgetful too.

You can cope by making certain adjustments. For example, when you're looking for your eyeglasses and can't find them in the obvious place, don't forget to check the freezer. Stock up on "Sorry, I forgot your birthday" cards.

Some of this behavior may be due to a lack of estrogen, which can be the cause of various minor ailments (headaches, joint pain, constipation, bladder problems and yeast infections) as well as depression, irritability, crying spells and fatigue. (In fact, some perimenopausal women who don't respond to antidepressants become more comfortable when their estrogen level is raised.) Hormones can give you some relief. So can taking good care of yourself.

**A good doctor can help you figure out whether you feel crummy because of true depression, a hormone deficiency or too much chocolate and not enough walking.**

●

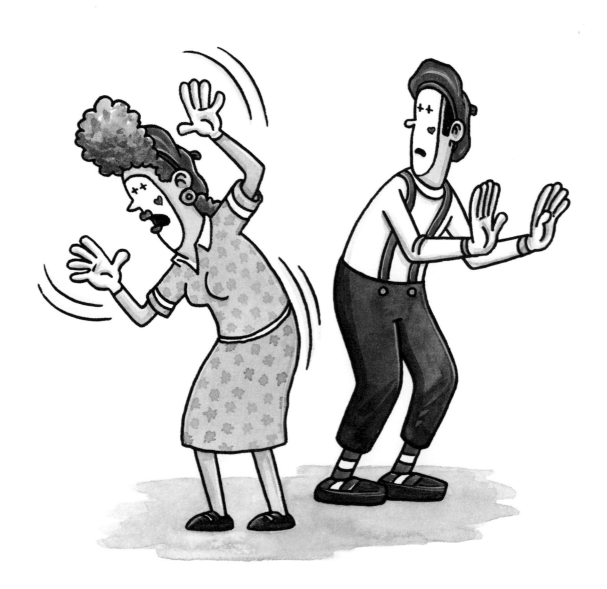

# "So my problems are all physiological? None of them are in my head?"

*S*ome of your strange menopausal behavior may indeed be psychological.

Though the overwhelming majority of women report that they never feel depressed as a symptom of menopause, it is just possible you may focus on the fact that at this stage of your life, you are more likely to suffer from progressive bone loss (osteoporosis); arteriosclerosis; drying of the vagina, bladder and skin; uterine and breast cancer; and heart attack. To keep your spirits up, try not to dwell on these things.

However, it is true that your spirits may be somewhat dampened at the prospect of seeing 50 — or 60 — candles on the next major cake.

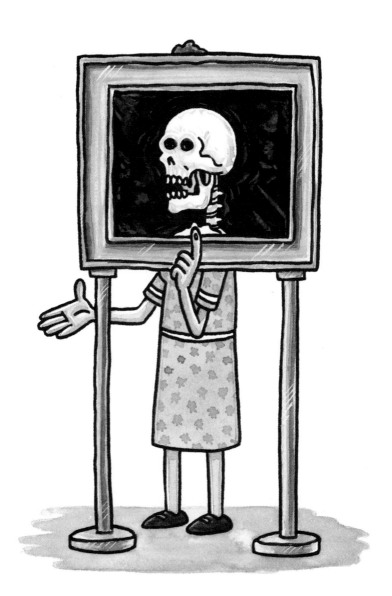

And it is also true that you are leaving your childbearing years. Your "babies" are leaving home, getting married or even having babies of their own.

Try this on for size: "Hi, Grandma."

Another thing: How's the hubby? Going through his own midlife crisis? Does he make you nervous by   a) talking of retiring soon, b) spending a lot of time looking at pictures of young girls who aren't his daughter,   c) wondering aloud how he'd look with his hair dyed?

Menopause isn't your only problem, but it does provide a good excuse and makes a suitable alternative from the usual scapegoats —

your mother, your husband or lack of one, your thighs — that you blame for whatever's wrong in your life.

It's certainly a much handier excuse than PMS, which only gets you off the hook for a day or two a month. Now, you can say things like, "Gee, I'd love to help, but I think I'm going to be out of it for the next couple of years."

And if you need an excuse to buy that hang glider, now's the time. Blame it on the big M.

. . . . . . . . . . . . . . . . . . . . . . . . . . . . . . . . . . . . . . . . . . . . . . . . . . . . . . . . . . . . .

# "What should I tell my doctor?"

*K*eep a gynecological "calendar" (when you last began to bleed, how long it lasted, how heavy was the flow, if you skipped) to bring to the gynecologist. (If you note, for example, that you get hot flashes after dinner, he may suggest you eliminate alcohol and/or caffeine.) Report any spotting. Report if you've been depressed. Don't forget to mention it if you've had trouble sleeping.

Doctors have begun to realize that the women who were thought to have gone crazy at menopause were probably just suffering from sleep disorders. Insomnia is a common symptom of menopause, but many women don't realize there is a connection. Knowing that there is can provide a great deal of relief.

**Some women say that shopping from catalogues in the middle of the night really helps. It's amazing what relief one call to an 800 number can provide.**

●

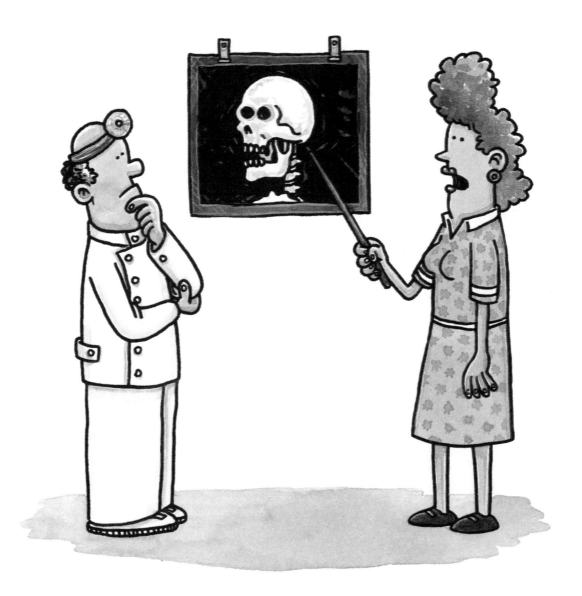

# "What should I tell my husband?"

*T*ell him only as much as you think he'd like to hear. (Most men are about as interested in the details of your menopause problems as you are in war movies. Remember this and don't expect a lot.)

It might be more useful to tell him what you'd like to hear. If he can't make it up, tell him to borrow ideas from the ads for hair dyes and wrinkle creams: "You're not getting older, you're getting better," that kind of thing.

Tell him you'd like to hear that he likes wrinkles (doesn't he like the California Raisins?) but that of course he doesn't notice any on you. Tell him to tell you that he's actually looking forward to the day when your breasts sag a little because it will be more comfortable to hug you — but of course (he should add) he doesn't see any sign of that yet.

Explain that you may be having some changes in mood. You may even be a bit forgetful, which could actually be a plus. Though you may not remember to pick up his shirts from the laundry, you will also forget the time he forgot to buy you a birthday present and what he did at the office party in 1968.

Reassure him that there is no reason for your sex life to go downhill after menopause — at least there is no reason that is linked to menopause.

Concentrate on the good news. Tell him how much money you will be saving on sanitary supplies. Remind him that he no longer has to explain why, though he's all for vasectomy as a concept, he doesn't feel it's appropriate in his case.

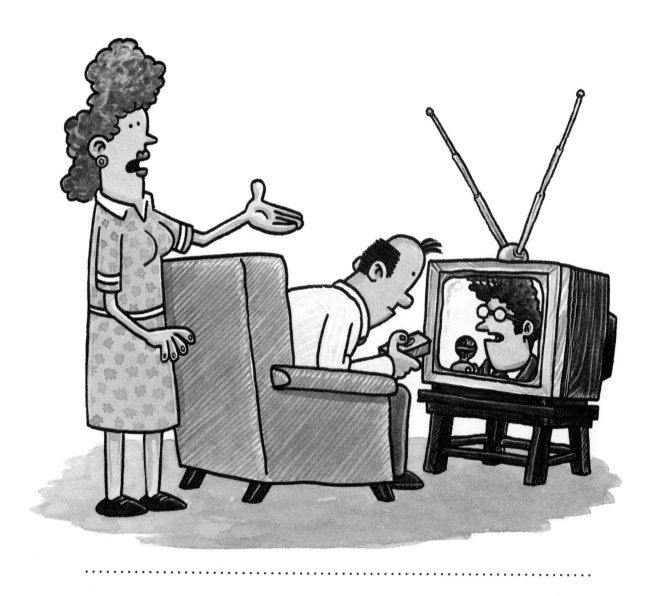

# "How long does this go on?"

*M*ale talk show hosts give the impression it happens overnight. Women who complain a lot make you think it never ends.

Actually, the process is gradual but not eternal. Changes in the ovarian function start in the mid-thirties for most women. While some experience symptoms of menopause for as long as fifteen years, most women experience the major symptoms for just a year or two. Less than a quarter of women have flashes for five years.

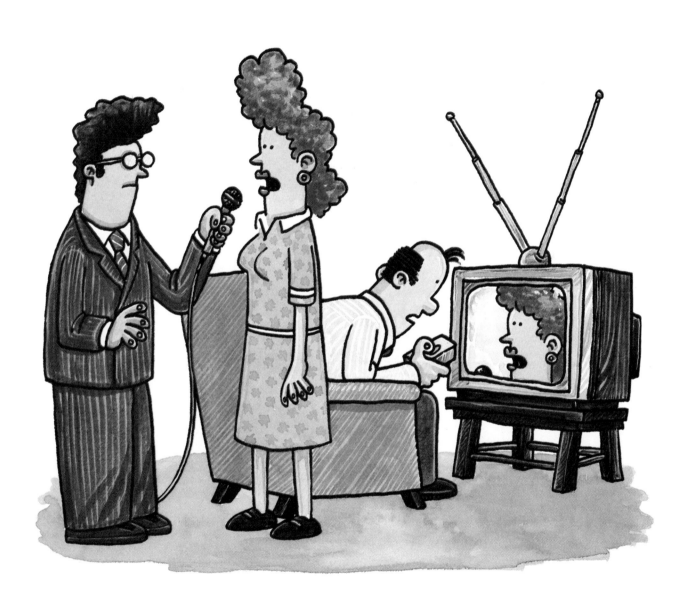

# "What happens to my sex life?"

Once estrogen levels decline, the quantity of vaginal secretions decreases and vaginal tissues become dryer. The mucous membrane lining of the vagina becomes thin and weaker. You may have itching, irritation, discharge and sometimes bleeding (though not usually until you're postmenopausal). Intercourse may become uncomfortable and irritating.

You may prefer simply to say you have a headache.

Alternatively, you can use an over-the-counter lubricant or prescription estrogen cream. The newest ones are very effective and long-lasting. To make yourself more comfortable, don't use personal hygiene sprays, which can irritate dry tissues. Since you're more vulnerable to infection, make sure to dry thoroughly after bathing, and wear cotton-crotch underwear and pantyhose. And avoid antihistamines, since they dry out all mucous membranes — not just the ones in your nose. Hormone replacement therapy, if you decide to use it, offers complete relief from this symptom, and others — such as fatigue and anxiety — that cause decreased interest in sex. Your lack of interest in sex may also be due to a decrease in testosterone, the male sex hormone that women's bodies produce in very small quantities. If you have a major loss of libido, your doctor can give you a little zip by prescribing some. (Just a little bit of testosterone, of course. You won't feel more womanly if you're growing a beard.)

Some women lose interest in sex just because they feel they're growing older and less attractive. (Though it may seem unkind to note, and it probably won't help, so is your husband. Who is he to criticize?) Now's the time for a makeover.

Doctors recommend having an active sex life because that keeps your vaginal walls elastic and helps make sex comfortable. Unfortunately, doctors are less useful at helping you make this happen. (To cure a boring sex life, no pill has been invented yet.)

You may be pleasantly surprised. Some women report that their sex lives improve postmenopausally, when there's no worry about getting pregnant. You can be spontaneous. You can "do it" on the spur of the moment and in unusual places. Of course, at this point it may take you a few more minutes to get into those places. You're not as flexible as you used to be.

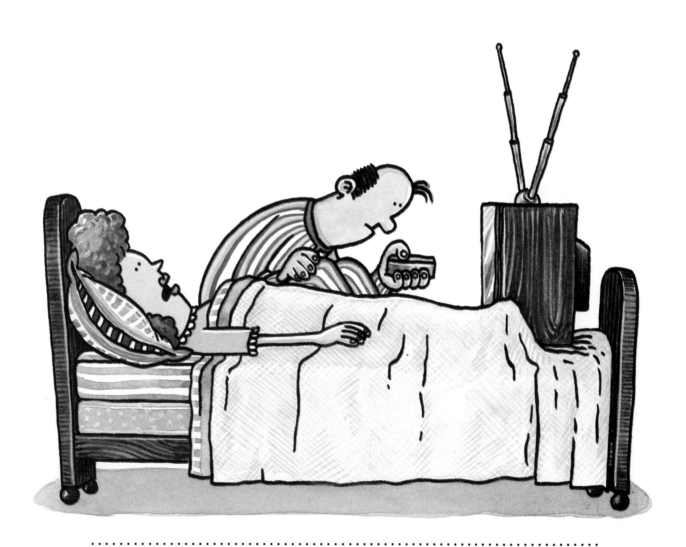

# "What's the story
## on hot flashes?"

*S*ince puberty, your body has become used to the presence of estrogen. Hot flashes seem to be linked to its withdrawal.

As the estrogen levels decline, the pituitary gland tries to stimulate the ovaries to make more of it with hormones that are released into the bloodstream in little bursts.

The bursts seem to create an instability in the mechanism that controls the blood vessels in the face, neck, chest and, sometimes, hands. They expand so much that blood rushes through them and causes the "flash."

It's a warm feeling, generally in the face, neck and chest, accompanied by a red flush and perspiration. It lasts from several seconds to several minutes and may come along with headaches, dizziness and/or nausea. Most of the time they occur less than once a day, but they may strike in rapid succession, just 10 to 30 minutes apart, or in the middle of the night. In fact, hot flashes are more common in the evening and night because that's when your pituitary is most active. Some women find it helpful to take a tepid bath before they go to sleep and to keep the temperature lower in the bedroom.

About 85 percent of all women have hot flashes. Three-quarters have them for more than a year but almost all for less than two. When in rare cases they persist, they're much less severe.

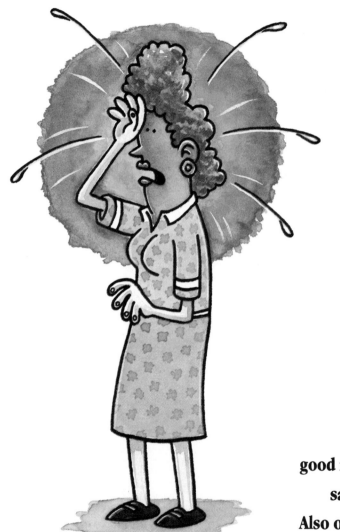

Here's the good news: You'll save on heat. Also on perfume. Warm skin helps radiate the scent.

# "Is there anything I can do to feel better?"

*J*ust because the side effects of menopause are considered "normal" doesn't mean you have to put up with them. You can minimize many of them just by following the general health rules you already know.

- Stop smoking. You probably started to smoke so you'd look older. That is no longer necessary. Besides, smoking weakens your bones, increases the possibility of heart disease and dries your skin.

- Stop drinking. Same as above, and bad for the weight besides.

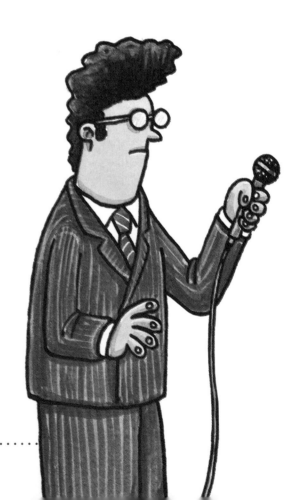

● Stay out of the sun and drink 6-8 glasses of water a day to help keep your skin moist.

● Unless you're eating milk products 2 or 3 times a day, take 1,000 mgs of calcium (with a meal) daily and 1,500 mgs when you're postmenopausal. (Though you may not be absorbing the calcium well if you're not taking estrogen, it can't hurt — unless you have a history of kidney stones.)

● Eat less caffeine, salt and concentrated carbohydrates to reduce the effects of stress on your body. Take 100 or 200 mgs of Vitamin B6* once or twice a day as a prophylactic measure.

● Taking 400 IU of vitamin E* twice a day might help with hot flashes.

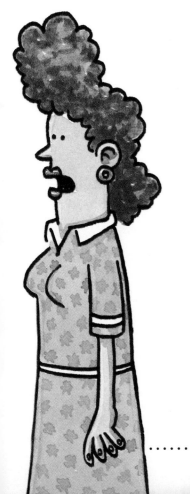

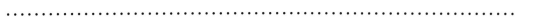
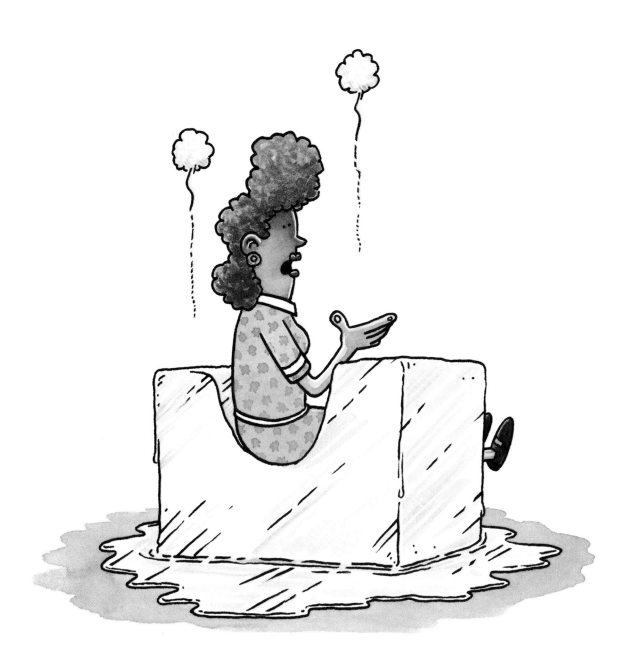

● Eat low-fat, low-cholesterol and high-fiber foods, lose excess weight and exercise to avoid heart disease.

● Cut down your eating, since (unrelated to menopause) your metabolism rate will begin to slow down at this point in your life. You'll worry less about aging if you look better. (Not everyone can manage this. Pass the bread.)

What do you mean, you're not having fun?

*Some doctors think 200 mgs of B6 and 600 units of E is the maximum. Check to see what your doctor recommends.

# "I've done everything I can. Is there anything anyone can do for me?"

*Y*ou're exercised, rested, eating little fat and all the fiber you can chew, swallowing all the water you can get down...in fact you're a paragon of healthy living. And you still feel lousy.

You can turn to your doctor for some medical help.

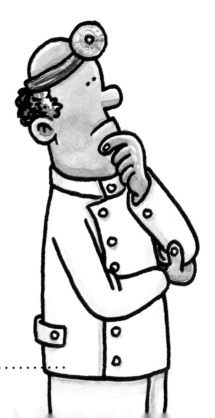

For excessive bleeding, progesterone alone may be the cure. But if the other symptoms of menopause are bothering you, the doctor may recommend a full course of hormone replacement therapy, or HRT. HRT consists of regular doses of estrogen accompanied by progesterone. Once you replace estrogen, all the symptoms of menopause disappear.

HRT has other benefits as well.

● It slows the process of bone loss. One out of three women are affected by postmenopausal osteoporosis, which leads to compression fractures (in the vertabrae) and long bone fractures (in hip and arm). Compression fractures may cause chronic, long-term pain, shrinking, even disfigurement (such as "dowager's hump"). Complications from long bone fractures carry a high risk of death. Calcium supplements and other

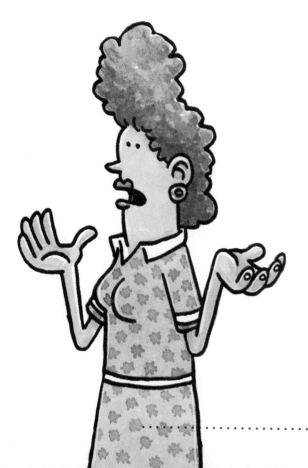

47

remedies are not nearly as effective as HRT.

- It reduces the incidence of urinary tract infections, which become a problem for many women once they are postmenopausal, and keeps the bladder in a healthier state. The same tissue that makes the vagina makes the bladder, and both the bladder and the muscles underneath it are sensitive to estrogen. If you have a stress incontinence problem (you urinate when you cough or sneeze), a little estrogen will help.

- It may keep the skin from aging and relieve arthritis joint pain.

- It has a beneficial effect on cholesterol levels and consequently on arteriosclerosis. Estrogen seems to increase the HDLs in blood (which is good), though progesterone increases the LDLs (which is bad). Still, on the whole, HRT seems to be more beneficial than not.

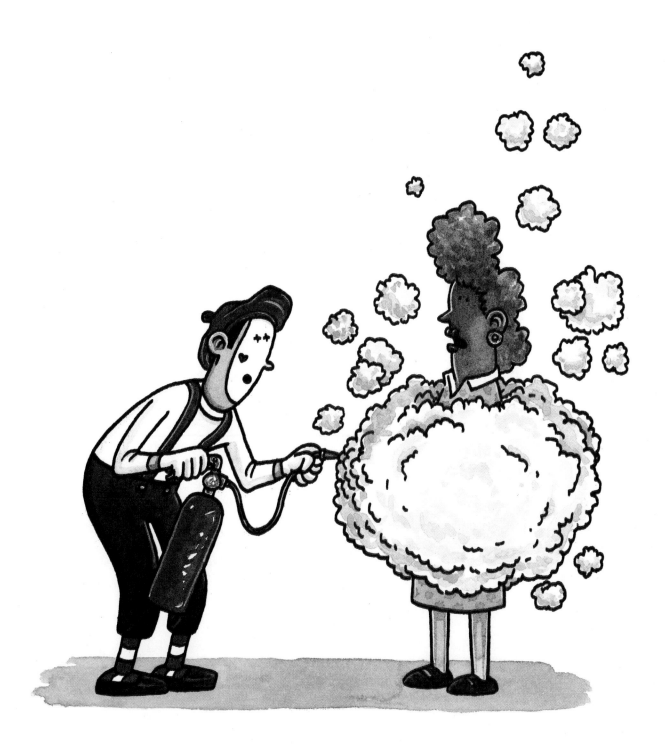

# "When can I start estrogen therapy?"

*I*n the past, HRT was generally begun a year after the last period, when it was definite that menopause had been reached. Otherwise, if a woman was spotting, doctors didn't know whether the cause was merely a light period or a symptom that had to be investigated.

A patient who is likely to get osteoporosis — if she is underweight or extremely slender, if she has a family history of the disease or if X-rays confirm she is at risk — may begin it in her 30's. HRT may be used preventively in the case of heart disease, too. But most women begin it just as soon as they are bothered by flashes.

Started early (during menopause), HRT will prevent irreversible changes in bones and blood vessels. Begun even many years after menopause, HRT may still have a helpful effect in preventing further bone loss and arteriosclerosis. And if a woman has had low-grade hot flashes for years and they begin to act up when she's in her 70's, HRT may be begun then.

**You didn't invest in that penny stock before it hit it big. You turned down the proposal from the guy who became a CEO in a Fortune 500 company. At least with HRT, you get a second chance.**

●

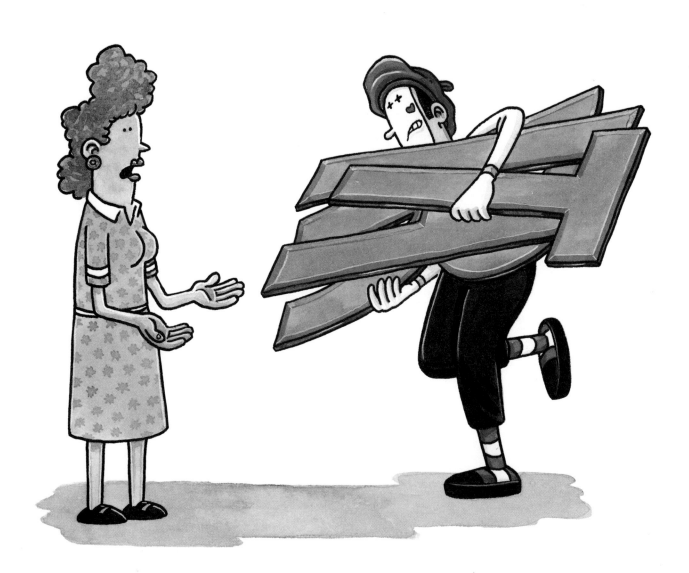

# "How do you take it?"

*I*t's usually given orally, sometimes as shots, and increasingly as transdermal patches, cellophane discs applied like a bandage strip twice a week.

The patches are convenient and administer estrogen directly into the bloodstream, but oral dosages may provide more benefits for cholesterol and osteoporosis. In any case, the progesterone must be taken orally.

Normal ovaries produce different amounts of estrogen daily, and prescribed dosages may vary, too. In the case of weight gain, bloat or unusually heavy bleeding, the dose may be reduced.

For the younger woman, higher doses are prescribed, since her body is used to the presence of a higher level of estrogen. A higher dose may be given in very hot weather, when hot flashes may be more frequent. At least in the summer everyone else is having hot flashes too.

**You used to have to remember to take your birth control pills. Now you have to remember to take your HRT medication.**

●

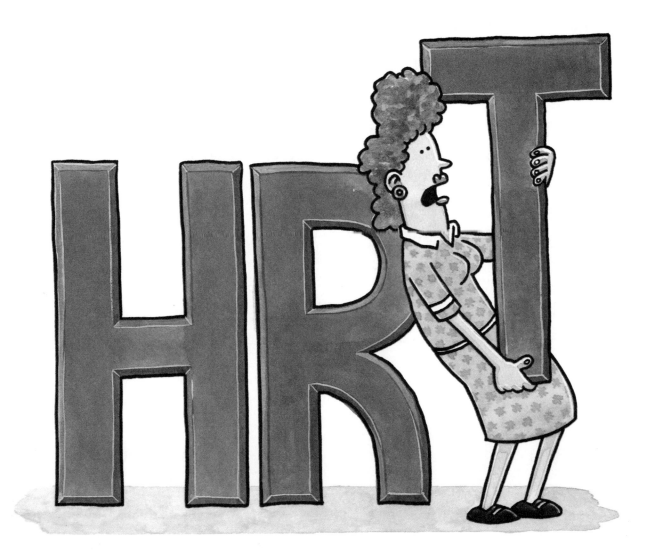

# "What are the risks with HRT?"

*T*o date, there doesn't seem to be an increased risk of breast cancer, though testing continues.

The likelihood of phlebitis and gall bladder disease increases.

HRT may make fibroids grow.

It's definitely not for you if you have known or suspected cancer of the breast or other estrogen-dependent cancer (such tumors may be stimulated to grow in the presence of estrogen); active blood-clotting problems; pregnancy; undiagnosed abnormal vaginal bleeding.

There are very few medical conditions with contraindications for HRT.

Make your decision about it after consulting with a doctor who is familiar with your medical background.

**If you have a hard time recalling your entire medical history, try a cousin whose specialty is disaster recall. There's usually one in every family.**

●

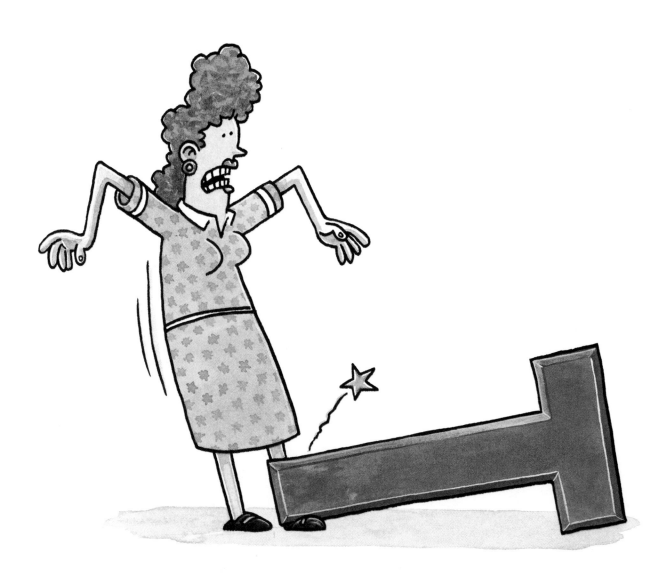

# "What are the
## negatives involved
## in using HRT?"

$Y$ears ago, estrogen was given without progesterone. That produced an increased — though still statistically very small — risk of cancer. When estrogen is administered with progesterone, the risk of uterine cancer appears to be the same as for the general population.

The presence of the progesterone initiates the "period" that is the cleaning out of the uterine lining. If you hate your period so much you can't wait to get rid of it, then HRT is not for you. But patience pays off. In most cases, the flow is light and the cycle is short, and the period usually fades out after two to three years. (At least you don't have to keep track of it. With no eggs, you can't get pregnant.)

Women who are extremely sensitive to the tiniest dosage of estrogen may find that their breasts become very tender. There are also rare reports

**You get to select whether
to have hot flashes or to prolong
your period. Freedom of choice
is wonderful, isn't it?**

●

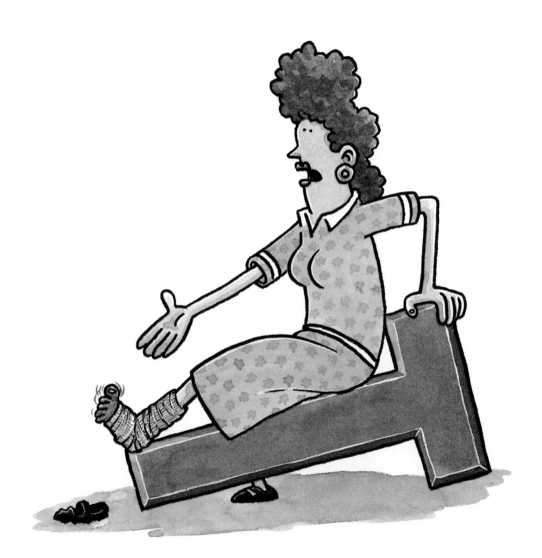

of queasiness, as in pregnancy, though in milder form, and some fluid retention. However, no major weight gain is linked to taking estrogen.

Some women experience headaches and moodiness. Slight pigmentation changes, such as the brown spots associated with pregnancy and birth control pill usage, may occur.

But having had problems with birth control pills doesn't mean you will have a problem with HRT. The pill uses synthetic estrogen. The estrogen you get in HRT is natural and in doses much smaller than in the pills or what your body would produce naturally.

Different dosages may relieve some of these problems.

You'll have time to find the one that's right. Hormone replacement therapy is ongoing. You can stay on it (unless there are counterindications) forever. While it continues, however, menopause does not.

# A final thought:
## Menopause
### is only
#### a temporary
##### condition.

*S*o, you may say, is labor, root canal
work and being stuck in a stalled elevator.
Well, you got through those, didn't you? It's possible that HRT will help
you through menopause with minimal problems. And if that isn't
the right choice for you, do keep in mind that menopause is a relatively

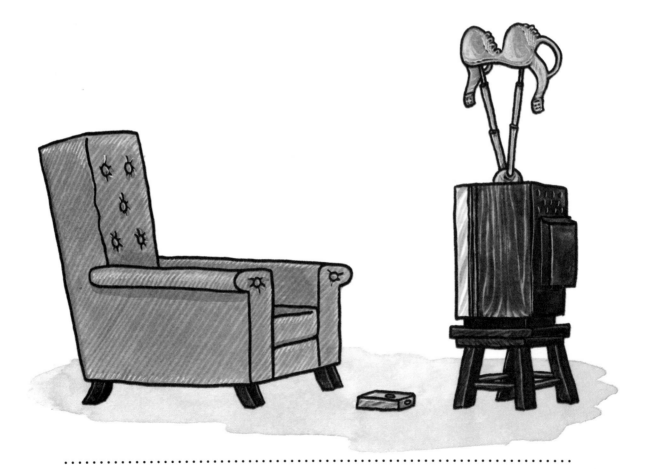

short event. You have many, many years — over half your adult lifetime — that you can look forward to. Take care of yourself and chances are you will enjoy them in good health. It's here at last: The chance to buy really nice lingerie.

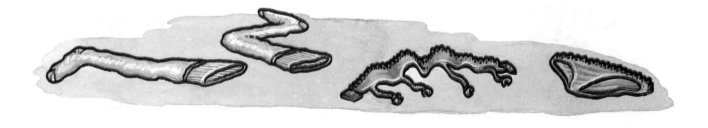

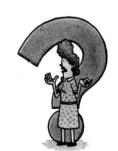

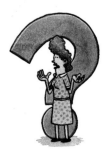

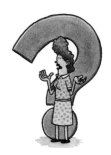
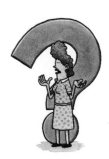
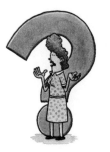